Home Remedies
For Eczema

Home Remedies For Eczema

By Monica Sidoine,
S.N.H.S. Dip. Herbalism

DISCLAIMER

This book is to serve as an informational guide for use in the home. The remedies and procedures contained in this book are meant to supplement and are not intended to be a substitute for professional medical care. Please seek a qualified medical practitioner for all ailments. The author nor distributors takes no responsibility for customers choosing to treat themselves. Your use of this information is at your own risk.

ISBN - 13: 978-1535012270
ISBN - 10: 1535012277

Proof Read by Jasmine Ned Anunda

Printed By Create Space Publishing
United States of America

ACKNOWLEDGMENTS

I would like to thank all those who have contributed in one way or another to the completion of HOME REMEDIES FOR ECZEMA.

I thank God for giving me the vision, wisdom and good health to write this book. For all he has done and will continue to do in my life.

For the many prayer warriors who interceded on behalf of this project and also their moral support.

I thank my daughter Jasmine Ned Anunda for proof reading.

Thank you all.

Monica Sidoine.

PREFACE

The procedures in this Book was designed to be as simple as possible so that anyone will be able to follow them. Most of the items used are local things which you would either have at home, in your kitchen garden or can be easily purchased from the local market or health store for a very low cost.

By using the simple remedies and health tips outlined in this book it should help you in your journey to recovery.

TABLE OF CONTENTS

ECZEMA

Eczema is an inflammation of the skin.

It can be chronic or acute. It is not contagious.

The symptoms are:
Rashes, itchiness, swelling, inflammation, blistering, irritation, reddening of the skin and the formation of scaly or crusty patches that may leak fluid.

It can affect different body parts such as the hands, face, ankles, back of knees, neck and upper chest.

Contact eczema is inflammation of the skin when it reacts to an irritant substance that it came in contact with. It is acute. It causes a red rash, blistered and swollen.

Atopic eczema is the most common type of eczema. It is chronic and affects persons with a family history of asthma or hay fever. It is most commonly seen in babies and children. It flares up every so often and then subsides. It causes the skin to be red and itchy.

Some causes are:
Radiation.
Stress, fatigue and sweating.
Bacteria, virus, parasites and toxins in the blood.
Genetic – children with a family history.
Environmental – exposure to dust, pollen, preservatives, detergents, soaps, perfumes, certain clothing and food allergies.

NATURAL REMEDIES

- Mix 2 tablespoons of aloe in a glass of water, juice or milk. Drink it twice daily.

- Steep 1oz of chamomile in 1 liter of boiling water for 30 minutes. Take 1 cup three times daily.

- Steep 1oz of strawberry leaves in 1 liter of boiling water for 30 minutes. Drink 1 cup 4 times daily.

- Steep 1oz plantain in 1 liter of boiling water for 30 minutes. Drink 1 cup three times daily.

- Steep 1oz of turmeric in 1 liter of boiling water for 20 minutes. Drink 1 cup 3 times daily.

- Steep 9 orange leaves in 1 liter of boiling water for 30 minutes. Take 1 cup three times daily.

- Steep 9 patchouli leaves in 1 liter of boiling water for 30 minutes. Take 1 cup three times daily.

- Steep 1oz of sarsaparilla root in 1 liter of boiling water for 30 minutes. Drink 5 cups daily before meals.

- Boil 2 tablespoons of red clover seeds in 1 liter of water for 30 minutes. Take 1 cup twice daily for two weeks.

- Steep 1 tablespoon of goldenseal in 2 cups of boiling water for 30 minutes.
  Take 1 cup twice daily for two weeks.

- Drink 1 glass of carrot juice twice daily.

- Drink 1 glass of cabbage juice daily.

- Drink I glass of orange juice twice daily.

- Drink at least 8-10 glasses of water daily.

- Eat 4 ½ lbs. of apples a day for 3 – 5 consecutive days. Water may be drunk. The apples may be eaten raw, as applesauce, baked or cooked but without additional sweeteners. This treatment may be repeated several times a year.

- Eat 3 cloves of raw garlic three times daily.

- Consume 2 tablespoons of flaxseed oil daily.

- Consume lots of raw carrots and cabbage; and green leafy vegetables.

- Consume yellow and orange fruits.

- Consume wheat germ, sesame, molasses, whole grains and bananas.

- Consume beans, peanuts and sunflower seeds.

- Consume vegetable juices such as watercress, cucumbers, asparagus and radish.

- Consume soy milk.

- Consume 4 tablespoons of coconut oil daily.

- Combine equal parts of honey and cinnamon into a paste.
  Apply it to the affected areas.
  Leave it on for 30 minutes. Rinse it off with warm water.
  Do it daily.

- Combine 2 tablespoons of powdered nutmeg and 2 teaspoons
  of olive oil into a paste.
  Apply it to the affected areas for 20 minutes. Rinse it off with
  cool water.
  Do it daily.

- Blend a cucumber with some water. Strain it.
  Apply it to the affected areas. Allow it to air dry.
  Rinse it off with warm water.
  Do it at least 3 times daily.

- Combine equal parts of apple cider vinegar and water.
  Apply it to the affected areas.

- Combine equal amounts of aloe and olive oil; add a few
  drops of vitamin E oil to it.
  Apply it to the area twice daily.

- Mix 4 teaspoons coconut oil, 10 drops patchouli essential oil
  and 2 drops wheat germ oil.
  Apply it to the area twice daily.

- Warm 2oz of almond oil and dissolve 2oz of cocoa butter in
  it. Remove it from the heat and mix till it gets like a paste.
  Apply it to the skin.

- Steep 1 tablespoon each of yarrow, yellow dock and burdock root in 2 ½ cups of boiling water for 30 minutes. Strain it. Add 1lb of cocoa butter to it. Put it on a low heat, stirring for a few minutes until it gets like a paste.
  Apply it to the area.

- Mix 2 teaspoons almond oil and 8 drops oregano essential oil.
  Apply it to the area 3 times daily.

- Mix 2 tablespoons of castor oil with 1 tablespoon of almond or coconut oil.
  Apply it gently to the skin.

- Mix 2 teaspoons coconut oil, 1 teaspoon almond oil, 8 drops sweet orange essential oil and 2 drops wheat germ oil.
  Apply it to the area twice daily.

- Mix 4 teaspoons of wheat germ oil with 8 drops of cedarwood essential oil.
  Apply it to the area 3 times daily.

- Warm coconut oil.
  Massage it onto the area at least 4-6 times daily.

- Avocado oil - Boil overripe avocados in a bowl of water. Scoop the oil out with a spoon. Strain through a muslin cloth. Massage the area with it.

- Mix 2 parts of olive oil and 1 part of lime water shaken together.
  Apply it 2-3 times daily in covered areas also after every hand washing for eczema on hands.

- Grind 1oz each of neem leaves and turmeric root. Add 2 tablespoons of coconut oil to make a paste.
  Apply it to the affected areas. Let it air dry and then rinse it off with warm water.
  Do it daily.

- Combine 1 ½ tablespoons of clay, 3 drops of benzoin and some water to make a smooth paste.
  Apply it to the affected areas for at least 20 minutes. Rinse it off with chamomile tea.
  If the condition is acute, repeated it at least 3 times daily.

- Mix 1 tablespoon of cold milk with 2 tablespoons of ground oats into a paste.
  Apply it over the affected areas for 15 minutes. Rinse off.
  Do it daily.

- Mix 1 tablespoon of powdered turmeric with some milk to make a smooth paste.
  Apply it to the affected areas for 20 minutes twice daily.
  Rinse off and wipe the area with a cloth or paper tissue dipped in vegetable oil to remove the paste.

- Steep 1oz of chamomile in 1 liter of boiling water for 15 minutes.
  Apply it to the area throughout the day or use it in the bath water.

- Steep 1oz of turmeric in 1 liter of boiling water for 20 minutes.
  Apply it to the area at least 3 times daily.

- Soda Alkaline Bath.

- Epsom Salt Bath.

- Charcoal Bath.
  Once or twice daily for an hour or two.

- Have a lukewarm Oat Bath daily.

- Boil 3oz of rosemary leaves in 1 liter of water. Steep for 20 minutes, strain.
  Apply it to the area or add to the bath.

- Take a Hot Foot Bath at 104-106 degrees for twenty minutes. If sweating occurs, take a shower at 65 degrees for 1 minute. Do not dry. Take ½ teaspoon of unscented Vaseline, rub it lightly and quickly between the palms to mix it the water to form a milky mixture. Spread it lightly and evenly over the eczema, moving the palm in the direction the skin lines go to avoid pulling open any microscopic cracks. Allow the skin to air dry. This treatment can also be done without the hotfoot bath but after having a shower.

- Steep 1oz of red clover or goldenseal in 1 liter of boiling water for 30 minutes. Cool.
  Use it as a Cold Compress to the area for 20 minutes four times a day.

See the Hydrotherapy Section for all of the Baths and the Cold Compress.

- Mix some goldenseal powder with some vitamin E oil.
  Put it on the affected area.

16

- If the eczema is located only on the hands do hot and cold hand baths. 3 minutes in the hot and 1 minute in the cold. Repeat 5 times.

- Garlic Poultice - Crush fresh garlic, add warm water and just enough flour to bind the garlic. Place it on a cloth then over the affected part.
It hurts when left on too long, as soon as it hurts remove it.

- Boiled Carrot Poultice.
Boil the carrot and mash it.
Apply it to the area.

- Watercress Poultice.
Crush some watercress and wrap it in a thin cotton cloth.
Put it on the area.

- Oatmeal Poultice.
Cook oatmeal, cool then place it in a soft cotton cloth.
Apply it over the affected areas and cover with a dry cloth.
Apply a heating pad or a warm cloth over it.

- Cocoa Poultice.
Roast 10 cocoa seeds and pound them very fine.
Apply it to the area after taking a warm bath.

- Castor Bean Leaf Poultice.
Take 12 fresh leaves and crush them.
Moisten with a little warm water.
Apply it to the areas.

- Psyllium Seed Poultice.

Mash the seeds and steep them for 1 hour.
Heat the seeds.
Apply the poultice to the affected area for 15 minutes three times daily.

- **For Anal Eczema.**
Boil 1oz of psyllium seeds in 1 liter of boiling water for 15 minutes. Allow it to get cold and strain it.
Use ½ cup of the fluid as an enema 3 times daily.

Information in regards to poultices

It can be applied between 2 layers of gauze or light cotton, then cover with a bandage.

The poultice should be large enough to cover the area being treated.

Change it nightly and daily or it can be left on for about 20 minutes. The one that you would put on in the morning, remove it in the night and put on a fresh one to leave on overnight to be changed in the morning.

After removing it wipe the area with a cold moist cloth.

Health Tips

- After bathing allow the skin to air dry or just pat lightly with a towel, do not rub the areas with the towel.

- Wear loose cotton clothes and only cotton undergarments.

- Only use white tissue paper.

- Reduce the salt and sugar intake.

- Avoid dairy products and white flour.

- Avoid fried foods.

- Do not consume food items which have raw eggs in them.

- Avoid pillows which are made out of feathers.

- Avoid skin irritants such as detergents, soaps, chemicals, abrasive clothing, extremes of temperature and humidity.

- Avoid using perfumed scented soaps or cleansers.

- Avoid wearing rubber gloves.

- Avoid using antiperspirants.

- Avoid bathing in very hot water.

HYDROTHERAPY TREATMENTS

CHARCOAL BATH

Procedure:

1. Put ½-1 cup of charcoal powder in a tub of lukewarm water. Soak in it once or twice daily for an hour or two.
2. Finish with a tepid shower using no soap and pat dry.

COLD COMPRESS

1. Dip a washcloth in a basin with ice and cold water. Squeeze out the excess water.
2. Fold and lay it on the area to be treated. Pieces of ice can be put in the fold.
3. Change the washcloth every 3 minutes wiping the area often with a cold cloth until relief is obtained.
4. Dry thoroughly at the end of the treatment. It can be applied to any part of the body especially the face, forehead and neck.

Contraindications:

Do not use if the person have sinus or pleurisy.
Do not use it on a chilled person.

EPSOM SALT BATH

Procedure:

1. Pour 1-2lb of Epsom salt into a tub of hot water.
2. While soaking in it for 30 minutes drink 2-3 cups of hot herbal tea.
3. Immediately after the bath rest and cover warmly so profuse sweating can begin.

HOT FOOT BATH

It is very good for headaches, colds, flu, coughs, congestion, nosebleed, earache, sinusitis, menstrual pains, fatigue, fever, pelvic cramps and congestion, prostate disorders, nervous tension, toothaches, backaches, infections, relaxation, stimulates circulation and warms the body.

Items needed:

1 bucket about quarter filled with hot water.
Small basin of ice water.
Large pan of very hot water.
2 washcloths for the head compress.
1 sheet and a blanket or 2 sheets.
1 hand towel for the neck.
1 bath towel.
1 bath mat.

Procedure:

1. Drape a blanket to completely cover a chair, then cover the blanket with a sheet.
2. Place a bucket ¼ filled with hot water on a bath mat in front of the chair.
3. Remove clothing, sit and wrap with the sheet, then the blanket.
4. Close all doors and windows.
5. Place the feet into the bucket and wrap the sheet and blanket around the bucket to avoid the circulation of air.
6. Wrap a hand towel around the neck to hold the sheet and blanket in place.
7. Apply a cold compress to the forehead, changing it every 3 minutes.
8. Maintain the water temperature in the bucket by adding more hot water continuously by pushing the persons feet to one side and placing your hands as a shield between the feet and the flow of hot water.
9. Continue adding the hot water for 20-30 minutes or an hour if needed. When sweating begins give the person water to drink at intervals throughout the treatment.
10. At the end of the treatment lift the feet up and pour cold water over them very quickly, dry and put on warm socks. Unwrap and dry the body. Dress, cover warmly and rest for 30-60 minutes. Take a cool shower.

A heating pad placed on the lower abdomen and upper thighs or a heating compress on the feet repeated every 4 hours can be used to replace the hot foot bath.

N.B. Do not use this treatment for persons with diabetes, loss of feelings, unconscious, arteriosclerosis, elevated pulse.

OAT BATH

Procedure:

1. Grind 1 cup of rolled oats very fine, stir it into a full bath tub of warm water.
2. Sit in it for 30 minutes pouring the water over the entire body.
3. Stand in the tub and allow the water to drip from the body then pat the skin dry

SODA ALKALINE BATH

Procedure:

1. Fill a bath tub with water not too warm or too cool. Add 1 cup of baking soda or sodium bicarbonate.
2. Sit in the tub, dip and pour the water over the entire body for 30-60 minutes.
3. Stand in the tub and allow the water to drip from the body then pat the skin dry.
   Do as needed.

Other Book Titles by the Same Author

Can be viewed at this link:
http://www.amazon.com/author/monicasidoine

Healing Poultices

The Top 20 Most Valuable Herbs

Home Remedies For Cancer

Home Remedies For Losing Weight

Home Remedies For Blood Pressure and Diabetes

Home Remedies For Headaches and Insomnia

Home Remedies For Sinusitis and Tonsillitis

Home Remedies For Constipation and Diarrhea

Home Remedies For Asthma and Bronchitis

Home Remedies For Dehydration and Vomiting

Home Remedies For Pneumonia and Tuberculosis

Home Remedies For Stress, Depression and Anxiety

Home Remedies For Dengue and Malaria

Home Remedies For Heart Attack and Strokes

Home Remedies For Colds, Fever and Sore Throat

NOTES

NOTES

NOTES

NOTES